Managing ADHD and ADD with Diet

A comprehensive guide on how to improve and manage ADHD with foods!

Table Of Contents

Introduction 1

Chapter 1: What is ADHD/ADD and ADHD Diet? 2

Chapter 2: Review on Dietary Interventions Used to Control ADHD 7

Chapter 3: Guidelines for Making an ADHD Diet 11

Chapter 4: Brain-Enhancing Foods and Dietary Methods 13

Chapter 5: Dietary Interventions Used to Manage ADHD 18

Chapter 6: What to Do? 22

Conclusion 23

Introduction

I want to thank you and congratulate you for downloading the book, "Managing ADHD and ADD with Diet".

This book contains helpful information about how diet can affect ADHD, and how you can use diet to improve your ADHD.

As you will soon realize, the use of diet to improve ADHD has been severely under-tested, and inconclusive. Many of the studies thus far show a strong link between diet and the severity of ADHD symptoms. However, not enough studies have been conducted to confirm these links.

The dietary changes suggested in this book are simple, and easy to implement. If anything, they will result in a healthier lifestyle. By giving these tips a go, you will not only improve your or your child's health, but also have a great chance of improving the ADHD symptoms that are present.

If you are looking for a way to improve ADHD from home, reduce the need for medication, and improve your or your child's overall health at the same time, then this is for you.

This book will explain to you all of tips and techniques that will allow you to successfully change your diet and begin improving your ADHD! What do you have to lose?

Thanks again for downloading this book, I hope you enjoy it!

Chapter 1:
What is ADHD/ADD and ADHD Diet?

Attention deficit hyperactive disorder (ADHD) is a chronic health problem consisting of persistent patterns of inattention and hyperactivity-impulsivity, which may hinder development or functioning. On the other hand, attention deficit disorder (ADD) has all these things in common with ADHD, except that it consists of more symptoms that are related to directed attention fatigue (DAF). ADHD/ADD can affect young children, teenagers, and in some cases can also continue to show symptoms until and through adulthood. It has been reported that 3-5 percent of children are suffering from this disorder.

A diet for ADHD can be used to improve the functions of the brain and reduce ADHD symptoms. Here is some diet-related info on ADHD that you should always keep in mind:

- "ADHD overall diets" is a term that encompasses the types of food an individual consumes on a daily basis. Certain diets can either help improve or aggravate ADHD symptoms. It is also possible that a person may not be eating enough of the kinds of food that can improve ADHD symptoms.

- ADHD dietary or nutritional supplements include additional nutrients, like vitamins and minerals. Taking these supplements makes up for the nutritional deficiencies in the diet known to aggravate symptoms of ADHD. It is assumed that the nutrients the body requires could not be sufficiently gained from diet alone.

- An ADHD elimination diet is all about avoiding the foods or food components known to trigger or aggravate symptoms. It is assumed that the person ingests types of food that are not healthy and bring about adverse behaviors. A person's diet per se is not the major factor that triggers the numerous cognitive and behavioral symptoms observed in individuals with ADHD. However, a number of studies are looking further into the possibility that some types of food and food additives may impact certain symptoms in children suffering from ADHD.

Some experts believe there is a need to further investigate certain extreme diets such as the Feingold diet. For most children diagnosed with ADHD, this diet involves taking away almost all processed foods and some varieties of vegetables and fruits. It can be challenging to identify the number of children who may possibly be helped by diets that prescribe certain foods. In addition, many remain unsure whether moderate changes in the diet can be beneficial to conventional multimodal treatment. This includes behavioral therapy, psychotherapy, pharmaceutical intervention, support from the school, and educating the parents.

It may seem that there have not been enough scientific investigations and studies on the subject of ADHD diets thus far. Nevertheless, a lot of health specialists are convinced that diet may possibly help in managing the symptoms of ADHD. Anything beneficial to the brain may also help in improving ADHD symptoms. Although there is not a large amount of scientific backing for ADHD diets, many people have noticed positive changes in their children's conditions by manipulating their diet. It can be a cheap and effective way to improve a child's condition, with or without the accompaniment of medication.

Here are some dietary recommendations to help regulate ADHD symptoms in children:

- **High protein diet**

This may include eggs, beans, meat, nuts, and cheese. Choose protein-laden foods for breakfast, as well as during snacks in the afternoon. Doing this can help enhance attention, focus, and possibly lengthen the duration of effectiveness of ADHD medicines.

- **Omega-3 fatty acids**

Omega-3 fatty acids are sourced from coldwater fatty fish (like salmon), Brazil nuts, walnuts, canola, and olive oil. These may also be taken in the form of supplements.

- **Add more complex carbohydrates**

These include vegetables and fruits, particularly pears, grapefruit, tangerines, oranges, kiwi fruits, and apples. It has been found that ingesting complex carbohydrates during dinner can help improve sleep.

- **Limit intake of simple carbohydrates**

Simple carbohydrates include honey, candies, sugar, corn syrup, white rice, peeled potatoes, and food products made using white flour (like bread).

Control of ADHD symptoms through diet

Controlling ADHD through diet is more about the way a person eats rather than what they actually eat. The majority of nutritional issues among adults who have these conditions are caused by poor planning and being impulsive. The objective is to be more watchful of one's eating behaviors. It is imperative to plan and shop for ingredients that can be used to make healthier dishes. It's also crucial to know when it's appropriate to eat, and when to prepare meals ahead to avoid getting hungry. Make sure to have healthy snack choices available, to avoid opting for unhealthy food.

- Eat meals or snacks every three hours. Lots of individuals with ADHD/ADD eat irregularly. They can usually last for hours without eating and when they get hungry, will simply order fast food or eat whatever is close by. This kind of eating behavior is not beneficial for any person's physiological or emotional wellbeing. It can also trigger or aggravate ADD/ADHD symptoms.

- Adequate amounts of iron, zinc, and magnesium must be in the diet. Taking supplements or multivitamins can help maintain sufficient levels of these minerals in the body.

- Just enough complex carbohydrates and proteins can improve alertness, and at the same time can help diminish hyperactivity. These kinds of food can also provide adequate energy for daily activities.

- An increasing number of studies indicate that omega-3 fatty acids help enhance attention and concentration of individuals with ADD/ADHD. Aside from taking supplements, sources of omega-3 include coldwater oily fish, fortified eggs, and fortified milk. Two major types of omega-3 fatty acids that can be sourced from fish oil include eicosapentaenoic acid (EPA) and docosahexaenoic acid (DHA). These types of omega-3 fatty acids, even in supplement form, have been found to be beneficial in reducing ADD/ADHD symptoms. Supplements should have at least two to three times the amount of EPA to DHA to be effective.

New research indicates that children with ADHD have low levels of omega-3 fatty acids in their blood. Practitioners now recommend that children who have ADHD take omega-3 fatty acid supplements. Studies that involved placebos demonstrated that there was a minor but notable improvement in the behavior of those who took omega-3 supplements over the ones given placebos.

Chapter 2:
Review on Dietary Interventions Used to Control ADHD

In the last few years, using diet to combat ADHD (among adults and young kids) has intrigued many in the scientific community. Researchers have associated diet and nutrition to certain mental health conditions, particularly the development of ADHD in individuals. According to research studies, people with this disorder may be suffering from lack of vitamins and minerals, specifically omega-3 fatty acids. A researcher observed that the ADHD symptoms of a patient declined after taking a daily dose of nutritional supplements. However, that kind of benefit has not been completely substantiated, data-wise.

Science experts have asserted that many of today's children consume regular meals that consist of refined sugars and additives, like sweeteners, preservatives, and glazing agents, among others. This kind of diet can lead to allergies and problems in metabolizing fatty acids, which in turn may also have unfavorable effects on behavior. No conclusive evidence has been established showing that food additives can bring about symptoms of ADHD; however, there is definitive proof indicating that omega-3 fatty acids have significant effects on the learning capacity and behavior of children. Omega-3 fatty acids may be sourced from linseeds, flaxseeds, and fatty fish, like mackerel, salmon, herring, sardine, and anchovy. Omega-3 fatty acids are synthesized into docosahexaenoic acid (DHA) and utilized in the different organs of the body, specifically the eyes and brain.

More and more clinical trials are being conducted to look into the connection between omega-3 fatty acids and managing

ADHD. The use of nutritive or dietary supplements has been reported to produce beneficial results, however this has little scientific backing just yet. Researchers assert that without the proper amounts of omega-3 fatty acids in the body, the functions of the brain will be gravely affected. This deficiency can lead into the development of ADHD or aggravate its symptoms.

Studies were also carried out involving minerals, like zinc and iron, as well as sensitivity to different kinds of food. There are children with ADHD who were found to be deficient in iron. This mineral is essential for the brain to function well and people suffering from iron-deficiency anemia may have symptoms that include fatigue, depression, and apathy. However, scientific trials using iron supplements need further investigation. On the other hand, a study indicated that zinc supplements may be greatly effective in managing ADHD, however once again there have not been enough trials to positively confirm this.

The daily diet of some individuals comprises mostly of sweetened or carbonated beverages and commercially prepared or tertiary processed foods. This kind of dietary habit can cause blood sugar to go up and down, and can lead to episodes of hyperactivity. In some studies, researchers have found that intake of sugar may be associated with hyperactivity; however, more meticulous experimental studies do not indicate any connection. The issue of food additives possibly causing hyperactivity has gone through various deliberations for more than three decades. In general, studies have not supported the theory of food additives being associated with ADHD; nevertheless, there have been a number of clinical trials which have indicated slight effects.

A study seven years ago pointed out that sodium benzoate, which is a preservative, may intensify hyperactivity among children. Researchers assert that the results from their study show an unfavorable effect on kids between the ages of three to nine years old. The researchers do not imply that food additives cause the development of ADHD, but the UK government body responsible for food safety and hygiene suggests that parents try to completely remove or reduce food colorings from the diet of children who show signs of hyperactivity. Other types of food additives are yet to be tested to determine if they bring about the same effects.

Adults with ADHD can also benefit from most of the research and studies conducted regarding the diet of children who have ADHD. A study in 2005 indicated that omega-3 supplements helped to improve the attention span and focus of adults also. This is most likely because of the beneficial effects of omega-3 fatty acids on the central nervous system (CNS). A trial study which made use of essential fatty acid supplements showed that the antisocial behavior of adult detainees was significantly reduced.

A review of medical research found that sufficient levels of blood glucose among adult individuals helps in managing attention span. Difficulties in maintaining self-control are more probable to occur if there are insufficient amounts of glucose in the body. Hormones in the body may be responsible in regulating the amount of glucose in the blood, but there are also other factors that affect blood glucose levels. These include failure to consume appropriate amounts of food for long periods, alcohol intake, rigorous exercise, illness or infection, steroids, and stress hormones.

In the treatment of ADHD, the initial action plan is to accomplish a proper medical diagnosis and then consider and discuss all feasible options for treatment. Medical practitioners will be able to recommend medications that are most suitable for your particular situation. However, it is the patients who decide if they want to modify their diet.

Whilst there is not a whole lot of conclusive evidence to support diet improving ADHD just yet, there certainly are a few instances where it has been shown to help. Increasing the amount of Omega 3 in the diet, removing processed foods and artificial additives, and adding vitamin and mineral supplements such as zinc and iron will have no ill-effect on the person, and may improve their ADHD. So, there really is nothing to lose in giving a new diet a try.

Of course, as with any treatment this must be done under the supervision of a medical practitioner.

Chapter 3:
Guidelines for Making an ADHD Diet

It shouldn't be too difficult to make your child's diet ADHD friendly. Initially, you have to make certain to consult the physician who's treating the condition. This is very important since your doctor is the most capable person to determine if the modifications you want will be effective and beneficial for your child. The physician may recommend certain diagnostic exams to determine how well the brain functions. With your physician's help, you can make healthier decisions concerning diet modifications, leading to much better outcomes.

A medical practitioner is not only the most qualified to supervise the changes in diet and to make sure they are really beneficial. There are also nutritional or dietary supplements that can only be obtained through a doctor's prescription. It is vital to determine and monitor the dosage of any supplement conscientiously. Once you have consulted your doctor, you are ready to go! With their assistance, you can begin altering your child's diet. In this process, consider these tips:

- Do gradual dietary modifications. This can help you easily determine if each dietary change is beneficial or not.

- Stick to the diet for an appropriate period, like a month or so, to be able to ascertain any change or benefit. If after this time the diet modification seems ineffective, try another.

- In this process, it is vital to keep a journal of the modifications, as well as of the effects. For every change in the diet, indicate the time and date this was made, and also write down the effects observed. Presenting this journal to your attending physician during consultations can be greatly advantageous in treating ADHD.

- Take note that no type of food, diet regimen, or nutritional supplement has been medically verified to treat ADHD. Nevertheless, it is greatly beneficial to a person's general health, particularly of the brain, to stick to a good diet.

To make an ADHD diet more effective, consider the following:

- It is imperative to take ADHD medications as prescribed;

- Get seven to eight hours of sleep every night;

- Work out three to four times per week; and

- Learn relaxation techniques to improve attention and focus.

Bear in mind that by setting aside more time to understand your health and condition, you gain the opportunity to effectively identify which changes and treatment methods are most beneficial. Eventually, you will be able to point out which types of food, food additives, and nutritional supplements affect your ADHD symptoms positively or negatively in your particular case.

Chapter 4:
Brain-Enhancing Foods and Dietary Methods

Experts say there is no absolute treatment for ADHD through diet; however, foods that boost the functioning of the brain have been shown to have favorable effects on managing the symptoms of ADHD. In addition, patients who consume nutritious, balanced meals observed that their prescription medications have become more effective in managing their symptoms.

- **Caffeine**

It may seem contradictory since very effective treatments for ADHD include stimulants, such as methylphenidate. This is a strong stimulant that affects the central nervous system (CNS). The effects of a stimulant may not be the same for every individual with ADHD, but generally it helps them stay still and concentrated. Hence, some experts recommend caffeine in treating symptoms of this condition. Caffeine that comes from coffee, cocoa, and tea is a natural energy booster.

Caffeine has been known to be very effective in increasing one's energy and diminishing tiredness. It can also heighten one's alertness when accomplishing activities that entail concentration and focus. Current research indicates that caffeine can potentially work as a supplement that individuals with ADHD can take. However keep in mind that caffeine won't have the same effect on everyone. Trial it for a while and if it doesn't work for you, eliminate it.

- **Evidence-based research that involved animals**

Research findings show that brains of animals that were purposely modified to trigger effects similar to ADHD symptoms acted positively in response to caffeine. Animals that were given caffeine showed more attention over those that were not given caffeine. A previous study reported that giving caffeine to animals that manifested symptoms similar to ADHD prior the tests resulted in better spatial learning. This type of learning is mainly about the capacity to retain information regarding one's surroundings.

One example is a laboratory mouse that learns about the ins and outs of a maze. Among humans, spatial learning makes it possible for an individual to efficiently find their way amidst intersecting city streets.

- **Evidence-based research that involved humans**

Only a few clinical studies investigated the use of caffeine to manage ADHD symptoms among young children. Researchers of a study determined many years ago asserted that objective measures of hyperactivity showed decline after the kids took 300 to 600 milligrams of caffeine. Higher amounts of caffeine appeared to notably manage hyperactivity among the children. However, certain side-effects were also observed. Outcomes were the same among children with ADHD who were given amphetamine.

It would seem that caffeine as an optional treatment in the control of ADHD is lacking recognition and has not been fully explored. Further study may be necessary. However, for now caffeine seems to be extremely effective, whether used alone or combined with other stimulant medications. It can also help in lowering the dose of psychostimulants needed to have beneficial effects. However, no adequate data is available to endorse caffeine as a treatment for ADHD among children, so it is vital you consult your physician before adding caffeine to your child's diet.

- **Sugar**

For many years, a lot of prolonged opposing conjectures have continued over the idea that sugar causes children to be hyperactive. Many parents have reported that whenever their kids take in sugar, whether from beverages, candies, or pastries, they become restless and unmanageable. In truth, no study ever found a significant link between ADHD symptoms and consumption of sugar. However, it can be beneficial to reduce sugar intake to maintain overall health and to lessen any chance of triggering or aggravating ADHD symptoms.

According to clinical studies, carbohydrates and processed sugars can significantly impact the level of activity of a child. Since these refined sugars can immediately reach the bloodstream, the result is an immediate rise in the levels of glucose in the blood. As the blood glucose levels go up, this is followed by an adrenaline rush, which can make a child show hyperactivity. As mentioned, no evidence has shown that a high-sugar diet can lead to ADHD; however they have been shown to induce hyperactivity, which could aggravate the ADHD symptoms.

A recent study has revealed that sugar may affect dopamine levels in the brain. Aside from regulating basic brain function, the neurotransmitter dopamine is responsible for the individual's energy, focus, and memory. Brains of persons with ADHD usually show signs of dopamine signaling alterations. In a recent study, parents of kids who ingested more sugar reported increased difficulty in making their kids sleep.

Another study conducted among Australian children indicated a significant connection between a child's diet and ADHD. It was concluded that a diet comprised of increased amounts of processed sugar, red meat, fats, and commercially-prepared food, was linked with developing ADHD, while eating healthy food was not. Another major study reported that preschool kids who were often fed unhealthy food products were notably more prone to becoming hyperactive when they reach school age.

The outcomes in the studies mentioned were worth exploring; however, it is not that easy to make definitive conclusions regarding the actual effects of ingesting sugar on ADHD because other dietary aspects should also be considered. Nevertheless, reducing the amount of sugar children take in has other beneficial effects to their overall health, so it is a worthwhile dietary change that you can make, regardless of if it truly improves a child's ADHD.

- **Dietary choline**

Choline is grouped among the B-complex vitamins. It is needed in the brain for synthesizing the neurotransmitter acetylcholine. Children should obtain choline from their diet to improve their cognition systems in the brain. Choline is a precursor of acetylcholine, which is essential for the functioning of the central nervous system (CNS). According to research findings, the metabolism of acetylcholine mediates a person's mood, memory, and intelligence.

However, there is no rigorously controlled test documentation available to substantiate that dietary choline is particularly beneficial in treating ADHD. Food sources of choline include egg yolk, liver and meats, soybean, cauliflower, tofu, whole grains, flaxseed, salmon, nuts, beets, lentils, whey, wheat germ, oranges, and bananas. Research indicates that other nutrients like methionine and B-vitamins, like vitamin B-9 folic acid, are essential in order to sustain the body's required amounts of choline. Methionine is an essential amino acid that may be sourced from meat, fish, eggs, seeds, and nuts.

Chapter 5:
Dietary Interventions Used to Manage ADHD

- **Elimination diet for ADHD: Feingold diet**

Dr. Ben Feingold, an allergist and pediatrician initiated this diet more than three decades ago. He claimed that the Feingold Diet can help in managing ADHD symptoms. This was founded on the idea that food additives can be detrimental to the nervous system of young kids who are prone to develop ADHD. He also presented his theory about the sensitivity of developing brains to certain chemicals found in food. This elimination diet takes out certain food additives from the diet, such as food coloring, artificial flavorings, preservatives, and artificial sweeteners.

- **Processes involved in the Feingold Diet**

Food items that make use of the restricted ingredients are taken out from the diet one at a time based on a prearranged timetable. The child's parents are supposed to record any symptom or behavioral change they may observe during the process. Restricted foods or ingredients may be provided again just to verify a possible association between them and the ADHD symptoms, like hyperactivity. If any symptom occurs again, the food must be totally removed from the diet. If no symptom was observed after reintroducing the food, this may be returned to the child's dietary regimen.

Although this diet was conceptualized many years ago, not all experts in medicine are convinced that it is effective. A number of physicians do not accept the possibility that ADHD may be managed solely through a modified diet. However, other doctors of medicine, as well as parents with favorable firsthand experience, are convinced of its effectiveness.

There are studies that demonstrate a connection between using food additives, like food colorings or dyes, and ADHD. It was six years ago when a major consumer advocacy group formally requested the U.S. Food and Drug Administration (USFDA) to prohibit some food dyes in the making of food products being sold on the market. There was increasing evidence that these substances caused hyperactivity in children who are predisposed to developing ADHD. It was only five years ago, that the administrative body of Britain considered this undertaking for the children's safety.

Some clinical experts may remain unconvinced with the effectiveness of the Feingold diet but lots of people vouch for its positive effects on their lives and their children. The choice is left in the hands of the patients and their doctors if they choose to try this approach. According to a report, fifty percent of ADHD patients experienced beneficial outcomes after modifying their diet. For parents and children who wish to try the diet method, it is important to do so under the supervision of a physician or an expert in diet and nutrition. This is to make certain that the patient being treated continues to receive the right amounts of nutrients that their body requires.

- **Gluten-free diet**

Gluten is a component of food found in oats, rye, wheat, and barley. It is used as a thickener, or in the making of different food products, like bread, pasta, pizza crust, and ice cream among others. In the past years, there has been a growing awareness of gluten intolerance and a rise in the autoimmune disorder called Celiac disease. Patients appear to have allergic reactions whenever they ingest food items laden with gluten. When patients with Celiac disease ingest gluten, they experience symptoms that have been found to be damaging to the inside layer of the small intestines.

Patients who have autoimmune reactions to gluten were found to experience various symptoms. These include gassiness, bloated feelings, pain in the abdomen, constipation, diarrhea, vomiting, appetite loss, and inexplicable loss of weight. Damage to the intestines may lead to an inability to absorb nutrients through the gastrointestinal tract. The patient may suffer from a lack of essential nutrients and this lowers the body's resistance to disease. The only acceptable treatment for these patients is to follow a permanent gluten-free diet.

Doctors theorized a probable connection of Celiac disease to certain disorders, like ADHD. These medical experts reported that numerous patients with Celiac disease who were not diagnosed to have ADHD manifested symptoms like hyperactivity. In addition, it was also reported that the symptoms waned as the patients started to avoid gluten.

When people with Celiac disease are not able to get sufficient amounts of tryptophan from their diet, this can result to lower levels of serotonin in the brain. When this happens, ADHD symptoms may occur. However, medical experts continue to have a difference of opinion when it comes to the theory of Celiac disease being linked to ADHD. Based on a German study, children with undiagnosed gluten sensitivity had positive reactions to gluten-free diet. They concluded that this kind of dietary approach can effectively manage their ADHD symptoms.

Celiac disease was previously thought to be uncommon. Recently, experts have found that an increasing number of individuals are sensitive to gluten. Nevertheless, the link between gluten and ADHD certainly needs further study. With the outcomes of new preliminary testing showing potential, it may be beneficial for parents with children who have ADHD to try the gluten-free diet.

To be gluten-free means to avoid food items with gluten, such as breads, pastries, soups, sauces, and condiments, among others. Despite the limited food options, it is important to make the right food choices to maintain the nutrition levels the body requires. It has been fortunate that numerous food outlets, including specialty restaurants, these days offer gluten-free products. However, in order to maintain this kind of diet, it entails commitment and regularity. Furthermore, it is necessary to consult the physician treating your (or your child's) ADHD before making dietary modifications.

Chapter 6:
What to Do?

Aside from choosing healthier foods and scheduling meals, daily doses of nutritional supplements may also be beneficial for people who have ADD/ADHD. The reason for this is that lots of young children, adolescents, and adults these days do not eat nutritionally balanced meals for different reasons. Furthermore, symptoms and causes of ADD/ADHD vary from one person to another. Remember, it is imperative that you consult a physician prior to taking nutritional supplements.

Dietary approaches that can help alleviate symptoms of ADHD are highly beneficial for individuals who have been suffering from this disorder. To date, these dietary methods and nutritional supplements still necessitate additional support from the medical community. Presently, experts all agree that children with ADHD are recommended to have a balanced diet comprised of vegetables, fruits, whole grains, protein sources, and healthy unsaturated fats. Patients are advised to supervise their children and limit the consumption of processed carbohydrates, saturated fats, and junk foods.

While there is a lack of scientific backing thus far, the majority of studies conducted suggest that diet can have a strong effect on ADHD. Whilst the suggested changes in this book may not 'cure' the condition, they could have a drastic effect on the severity of the symptoms, and the need for medication.

Conclusion

Thank you again for downloading this book!

I hope this book was able to help you learn more about ADHD and diet.

The next step is to put this information to use, and begin improving ADHD with the help of food!

Remember to always consult a physician before making any dietary change.

Slowly make changes to the diet, and note if differences occur. In no time you will know and understand what works in your particular case, and have a great chance of improving your or your child's ADHD!

Finally, if you enjoyed this book, please take the time to share your thoughts and post a review on Amazon. It'd be greatly appreciated!

Thank you and good luck!

www.ingramcontent.com/pod-product-compliance
Lightning Source LLC
LaVergne TN
LVHW021750060526
838200LV00052B/3572